The No-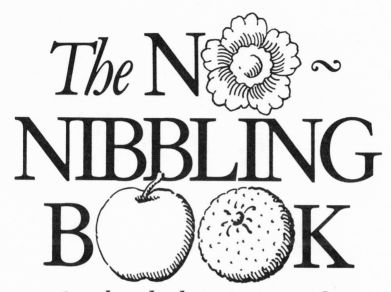NIBBLING BOOK

One hundred & twenty eight
things to remember or do at
the refrigerator door so you won't open it

ROBERT MARK ALTER

G. P. PUTNAM'S SONS, NEW YORK

You are trying to break an addiction, and you may need help. There is help for you in this book. There is help all around you. There are doctors, healers, counselors, therapists, clergy, family, and friends. Seek the help you need.

Library of Congress Cataloging in Publication Data

Alter, Robert Mark
  The no-nibbling book.

  1. Reducing—Psychological aspects. 2. Food habits—Psychological aspects. I. Title.
RM222.2.A454   613.2'5'019   80-24810
ISBN 0-399-12581-7

Printed in the United States of America

This book is dedicated
to the memory of my grandfather
Edward S. Simons
1891–1979

Mom and Dad, Gail and Milt, Yvette and
Irv . . . Another Place and Springhill . . .
Amethyst, Barbara, Barbara, Billy, Carol, David,
Diane, Donny, Gita, Harry, Jonny, Judith,
Karen, Katie, Lyra, Mary, Michael, Rick, Ruthie,
Samuel, Sandra, Sydney, Terry, Zea . . . David,
Marc, and Robbie . . . Thank you, friends.

Thank you, Connie. Thank you, Diane.

Jane and Greta. Thank you, God.

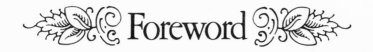# Foreword

At this moment you are standing at the refrigerator door. You are alone, and you are not hungry. You are about to open the refrigerator door and nibble.

You wish you weren't about to nibble, but you are, because you're addicted. You want to stop, and you can't stop. That's why you are reading this book.

This moment is a moment of choice for you. Do you or do you not open the refrigerator door and nibble? That is the question. *The No-Nibbling Book* is the answer.

In this book you will find one hundred and twenty-eight techniques to break the addiction called Nibbling. This addiction is also called Snacking, Noshing, Overeating, Compulsive Eating, Eating Between Meals, and Having the Munchies. All one hundred and twenty-eight techniques work. Some work sometimes, and others work other times. The last one works all the time.

Put a copy of *The No-Nibbling Book* next to your refrigerator. Put one in the breadbox, too. And put one in the car for your trips to the supermarket.

The No-Nibbling Book can be used to break any compulsion or addiction. It can be used to break the addiction to food, to sugar, to coffee, to alcohol, to cigarettes, and to drugs. At the bottom of all compulsions and addictions is fear. *The No-Nibbling Book* can be used to break the addiction to fear.

The No-Nibbling Book will not end your nibbling. You will. The book is an instrument. If you use it in the spirit in which it is offered, you can't fail.

But love yourself even if you do fail.

You won't fail.

That's the spirit in which this book is offered.

The Techniques

How to Read *The No-Nibbling Book*

Often; slowly; out loud; in a
gentle voice; to yourself;
to a friend; one page
at a time; as if you mean
business.

Ask yourself the following question: "Is the thing
I am about to do nibbling or eating?"

If it's all going by very fast and you feel frantic,
if you're doing it standing up,
if you feel you couldn't choose not to do it,
if you're not hungry,
if you *think* you're not hungry,
if you're not even asking yourself if you're hungry,
if there is lust in your eyes as you look at the
    food,
if you're repeatedly bringing your hand to your
    mouth while thinking of other things,
if you're at a party, a ballgame, a movie, or a
    television,
if you hope nobody is looking,
if you don't care anymore *what* you're doing,
if you're angry, scared, bored, rushed, tired,

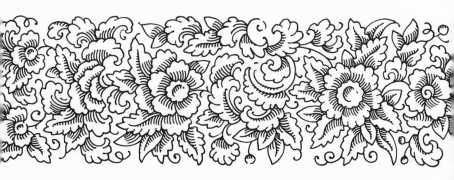

drunk, or stoned,

if you glanced at this book next to the refrigerator
and said, "Forget it,"

if any of these are true, you're nibbling.

If all of them are true, welcome to *The No-
Nibbling Book*.

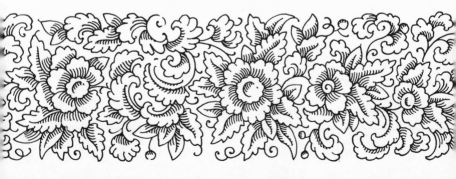

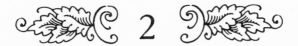

What's the big deal? It's only a little nibble.

Said Adam and Eve on their way out of the
Garden.

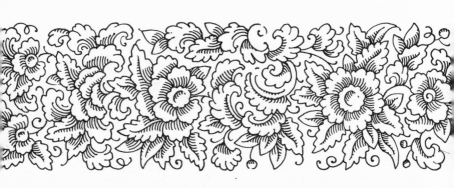

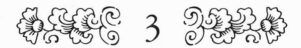

As you are standing at the refrigerator door about to nibble, say out loud, "I am standing at the refrigerator door about to nibble."

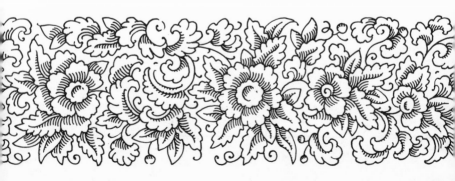

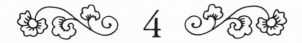

Become aware that you have a will by willing to do some small insignificant action, like touching your right forefinger exactly five times to the tip of your nose. Will to do that. Say, "I will touch my right forefinger exactly five times to the tip of my nose."

Now do it. Touch your right forefinger exactly five times to the tip of your nose.

You have a will.

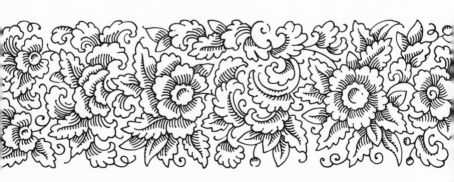

Where there's a will, there's a way.
You have a will.
Sit down right now and read all these pages.
This is the way.

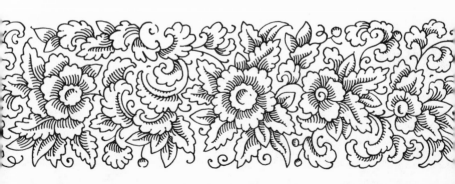

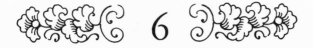

Your nibbling is a problem.
No, it isn't.
It's a challenge.
You *like* challenges.

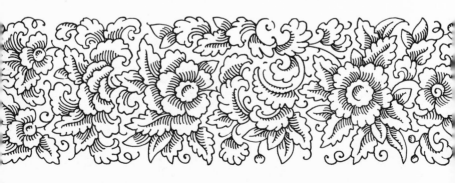

Once upon a time you felt fulfilled.

Then you were born.

Outside the body of your mother, you felt unfulfilled and your mouth began to move. You were searching for fulfillment with your mouth. Then you found it. It filled up your mouth and you felt fulfilled again.

Then you grew out of that.

One day your mouth was full and you didn't feel fulfilled anymore. You panicked. You rushed over to the refrigerator and tried to stuff your mouth fuller. You still felt unfulfilled.

You won't find the fulfillment you are looking for in your refrigerator. You'll find it in your life, if you look.

Step back from the refrigerator. Turn around.

Look at your life.

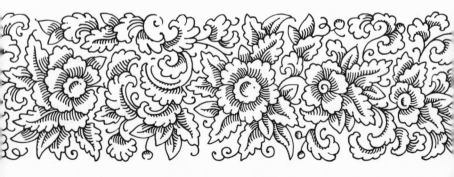

Breathe.

Keep breathing. Stand right there, don't move,
just keep breathing. Inhale . . . exhale . . . inhale
. . . exhale . . . follow your breath.

Keep breathing until the moment when there's
nothing else for you to do but walk away from the
refrigerator. Have faith that if you keep breathing
long enough, that moment will come.

Inhale . . . exhale . . .

Breathe.

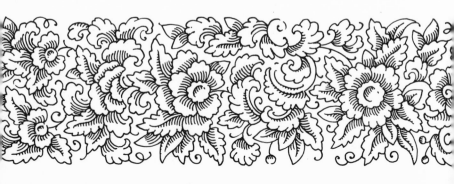

Ask yourself, "Am I hungry?"

If the answer is "No," don't nibble.
If the answer is "Yes," ask again.

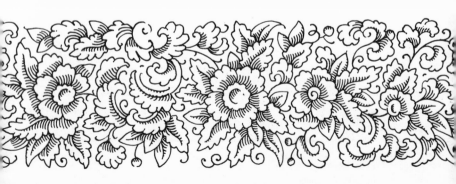

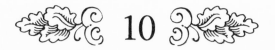

Your mind is like a computer. It is an absolute binary system, making billions of little yes/no choices every moment. Most of these choices are made below the level of your awareness, but right now, at this moment, with your hand on the handle of the refrigerator door, you are aware that you have a choice.

Yes or no.

Choose.

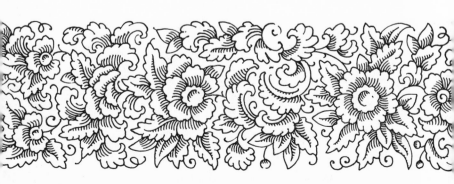

Listen to the excuse you're telling yourself this time:

> "Just this one. Then I'll get back to my work."
>
> "I haven't eaten all day."
>
> "I'm starving."
>
> "I've had a rough day."
>
> "I don't have time for a meal."
>
> "I'll get it together tomorrow. Today I'm going to be good to myself."
>
> "I feel great. One won't hurt."
>
> "I hate myself anyway, what the hell."
>
> "I can't let go of this habit. What'll I do without it?"
>
> "It's not time yet."
>
> "It's hopeless."
>
> "I'm beyond all this."

Listen politely to your excuse, but this time don't buy it.

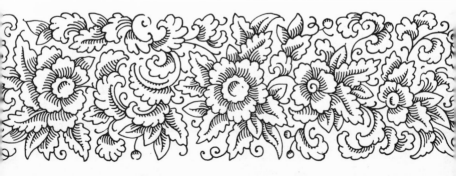

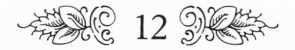

Consider the alternatives.

Get some fresh air. Find somebody to play with.
Go get a hug. Do work that you like. Take a
shower. Make love. Exercise. Meditate. Rest.

Assume that your need to nibble is one of these
needs wearing a mask.

Now take off the mask.

Are you confused about your eating?

What to eat? What not to eat? What time to eat?
How much to eat?

Your body is the governor of your state.

Accept the authority of your governor, and you
will not be confused.

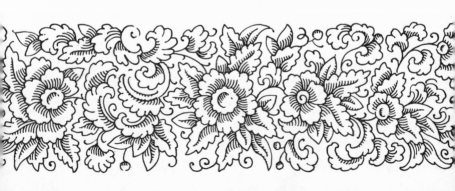

Bring your attention to your belly. Look down at it. Place your hands on it. Walk away from the refrigerator patting it.

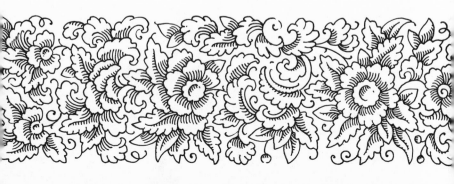

When you were a baby and you felt afraid or mad
or lonely or wet or uncomfortable for any reason,
you made certain noises, like whining and
whimpering and crying and screaming. Your
parents didn't like those noises, so they stuck
things in your mouth to shut you up. They stuck
breasts, bottles, pacifiers, and mostly food in your
mouth, and they didn't stop until you learned to
do it yourself. That's how you came to find
comfort in food.

Remember that you have been deeply, deeply
trained to put something in your mouth when you
don't feel good. It's not your fault.

But now you know, so begin to regain control
over yourself and undo the training. Begin to look
at your feelings. Stop throwing food on top of
your feelings. Create the conditions in your life
where you can express those feelings.

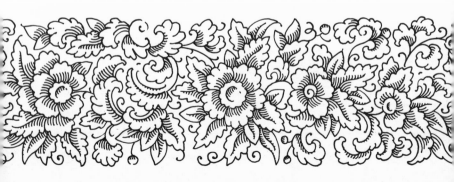

You are standing at the refrigerator door.

Close your eyes.

Imagine yourself stepping out of your body and going across the kitchen. From across the kitchen, stand quietly and watch yourself.

Don't judge. Just watch.

Watch what you're doing.

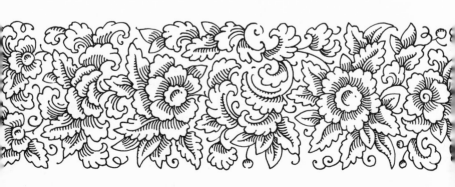

Bring your awareness into your body. Feel that you have a body. Feel that even though you are about to stuff food into your body, your body already feels stuffed. Your nose and sinuses are stuffed, your mouth is coated, and your throat is thick with phlegm. There is gas in your intestines, and your glands ache.

Ask yourself how could you possibly put another thing into this poor, congested body?

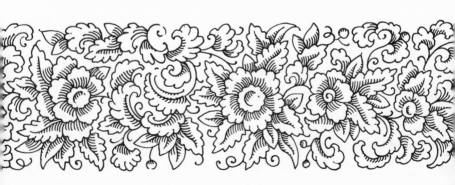

Become aware that you are frantic. Say out loud to yourself, "I am frantic." Remember that you are not to be trusted when you are frantic.

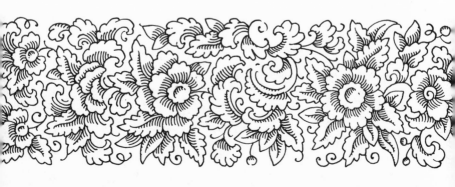

Remember that after this nibble you will feel pretty much the same as before this nibble, only slightly fuller, and mostly worse.

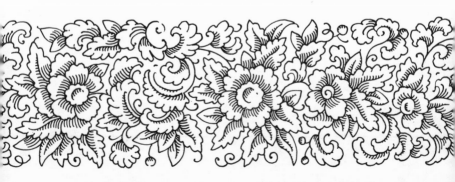

Listen to the voice of truth inside you. You know
this voice. You may call this voice the voice of
your higher self, the still small voice of your
conscience, the voice of inner knowledge, or the
voice of God. It always speaks the truth to you.
What is it telling you to do in this moment?

Listen.

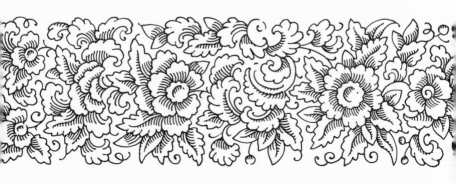

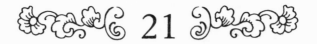

You do most of your nibbling standing up because
you're in such a panic to stuff food into your
mouth that you don't have time to sit down. So
sit down. Allow the panic to pass.

If it doesn't, and you get up again, sit down
again.

Keep doing this until you feel ridiculous, and then
leave the kitchen.

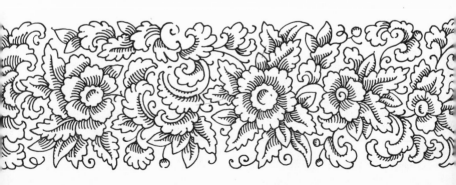

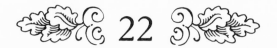

The feeling that you must put something into your mouth is overwhelming this time. Okay. That happens.

But remember that food, especially the kind and the amount of food that you are about to put into your mouth, is the worst thing you could put into your mouth, because it goes further than your mouth, all the way into your body.

So, if you absolutely need to put something into your mouth, consider the alternatives.

Consider your fingernails, your knuckles, your thumb, a friend's thumb, a toothpick, your moustache, or your hair. Consider anything that will go into the mouth and is not food.

Forget cigarettes. Avoid gum.

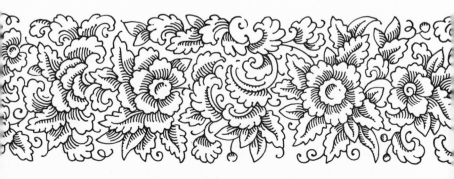

Close your eyes. In your mind's eye, picture yourself as a perfectly healthy person.

What does your perfectly healthy body look like? How do you feel?

In your mind's eye, begin to walk. How does it feel to be moving your perfectly healthy body? Run. Jump. How does that feel? Breathe. What does the breath feel like as it comes in and out of your perfectly healthy body?

Keep your eyes closed, and keep imagining yourself perfectly healthy.

Now imagine that you *want* to be perfectly healthy.

Now imagine that you *can* be perfectly healthy.

If you choose.

Now choose to be perfectly healthy.

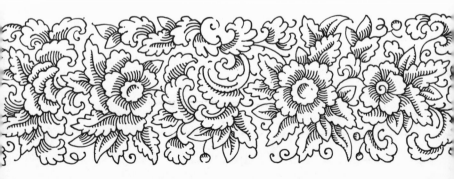

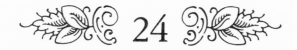

If you have absolutely decided to have this nibble, have it. But first close your eyes.

Now choose the number of mouthfuls you will have at this nibble. Listen for the number in your head. When you hear it, say the number out loud. Then subtract two. Say that number out loud. That's the number of mouthfuls you should have at this nibble. Then sit down and have them.

The awareness you will need to keep count, and to stop, transforms your nibbling into eating.

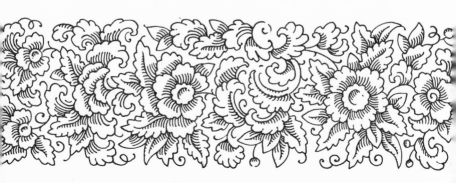

Say to yourself, "I don't have the will right now."

Now say to yourself, "Yes, I do. I just don't choose to employ it."

Now look at your choice.

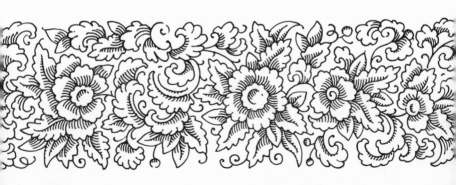

In your imagination, pre-taste the food you are about to nibble. Ask yourself, "Do I really want that taste in my mouth?" What taste *do* you want in your mouth? Do you want to change the taste in your mouth? One of the reasons you want to change the taste in your mouth is because your mouth tastes so bad from the last nibble you had. Go brush your teeth.

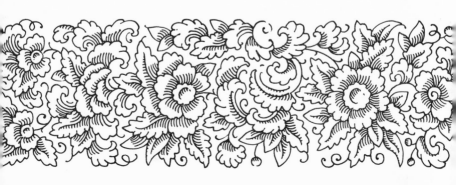

Don't open the refrigerator door this time. Walk away.

Now congratulate yourself. Feel very virtuous. Really pour it on. You deserve it.

Now realize that appreciating yourself feels better than stuffing your mouth with food.

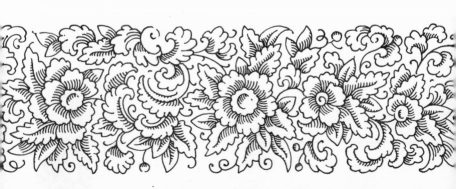

Close your eyes. Feel the compulsion. See it surge
against you again and again like waves from a
storm-tossed ocean. Just stand there, unmoved,
and hold your ground.

Stand.

You can stand it.

The storm will pass.

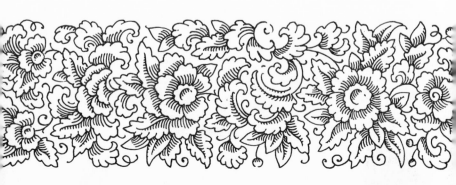

Pretend you're a cheerleader and do an inspiring cheer for yourself at the refrigerator. Stand on the sidelines and root for yourself like crazy. When you win, clap wildly.

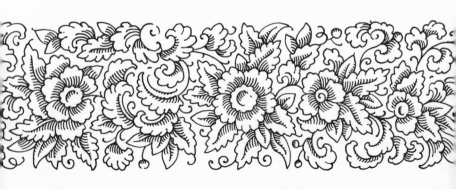

There are many small actions in the large action called Nibbling.

Walking to the Refrigerator. Opening the Door. Looking at the Food. Choosing the Food. Reaching for the Food. Grasping the Food. Preparing the Food. Bringing the Food to the Mouth. Opening the Mouth. Putting the Food in the Mouth. Chewing the Food. Swallowing the Food.

Within each of these small actions, there are smaller actions still.

You can bring your awareness and assert your will at any point in this process, but you have to be quick.

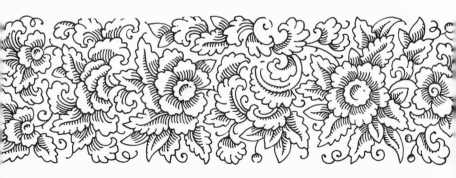

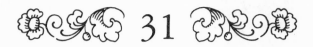

If you would take care of your body as you take care of the animal you ride on, you would be spared many serious ailments. For you will not find a person who would give too much hay to an animal, but the person measures the hay according to the animal's capacity. However, that same person will eat too much without measure and consideration.

You should eat only when justified by a feeling of hunger, when the stomach is clear and the mouth possesses sufficient saliva. Then you are really hungry.

Maimonides, *The Preservation of Youth*

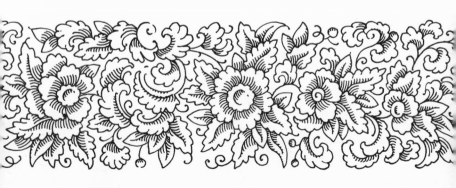

You're not hungry, you're thirsty.

Juice? Tea?

Water.

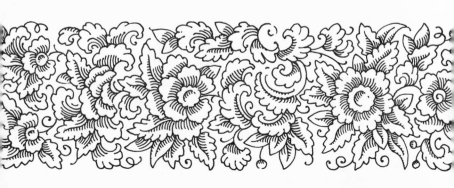

You are attached to your desire for food. You are also attached to your physical appearance. Not only do you feel hungry, you're vain. You want to look well. Your nibbling makes you look less well. You look pretty bad actually. At this moment, honor your vanity, bring it into your service, and allow it to stay your hand.

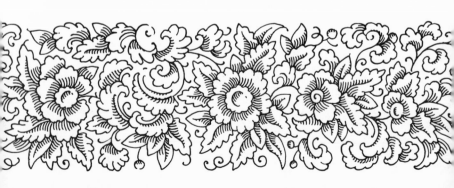

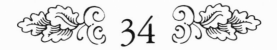

Close your eyes.

Become aware that you're not breathing.

Now take a deep breath and begin to breathe.

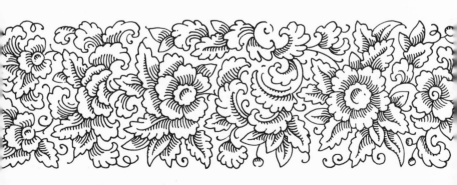

Declare No-Nibbling Days. These are holidays.
You celebrate these holidays by not nibbling, and
standing in awe of yourself.

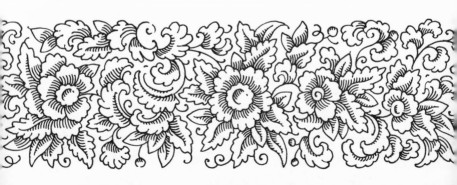

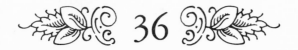

You're not hungry, you're tired. Your body needs energy. Nibbling pretends to give you energy, but actually it saps your energy. Consider the alternatives.

Lie down and rest. Do some yoga. Go for a walk. Take a run. Stretch your muscles. Soak up some sun. Do something pleasant. Read something inspiring. Meditate. Breathe. Yawn. Laugh.

These all give energy.

Of all the ways to give energy to a tired body, why persist in choosing the one way that doesn't work?

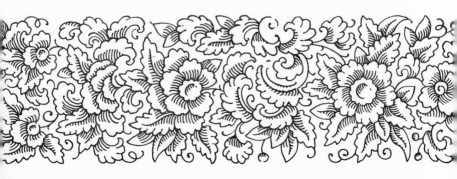

Your stomach seems to be calling for food, so you came over to the refrigerator.

Stop. Close your eyes. Bring your awareness into your stomach and visualize the kind and the amount of food that your stomach is calling for. See the picture. Then sit down and eat what you see in the picture, and not a thing more.

If you get no picture, your stomach isn't calling for food, it isn't calling for anything, you made a mistake, go away.

If you get many pictures of many foods, and they all start going by like a blur, your stomach isn't calling for food, it's calling for mercy.

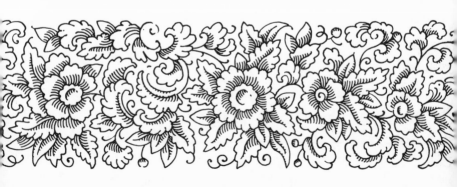

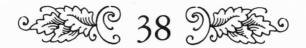

Actions have consequences.

Here are some of the possible consequences of the action you call Nibbling.

Stomachaches. Headaches. Hemorrhoids. Gas. Coughs. Colds. Bad breath. Bad dreams. Bad sex. Potbellies. Stiff joints. Pimples. Cavities. Worms. Wrinkles. Fat. Sloth. Depression. Cancer. Heart Disease. Senility. Death.

Read this list twice. First, as a list of plagues. Second, as a list of choices.

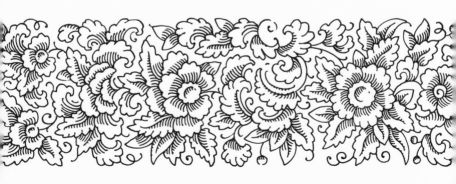

You are standing at the refrigerator door about to nibble. You are lost.

Say out loud, "I am lost."

Now turn around.

Imagine that someone just found you.

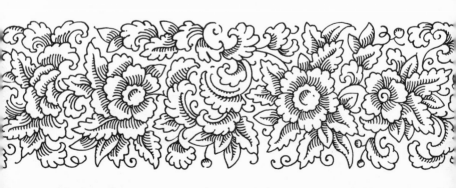

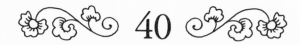

Close your eyes. Bring your awareness into your
body.

Somewhere in your body is the knowledge that it's
impossible for you to continue, you can't nibble
anymore. Search for that knowledge inside your
body. Search among all your aches and pains. It's
there somewhere. When you find the place where
the knowledge is, stay right there.

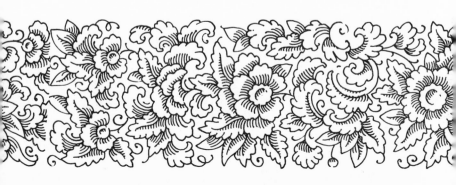

Your need to nibble is often your need to chew, which is usually your need to clench your jaw, which is what you do when you feel violent. You feel violent. It's okay to feel violent, but bring your violence some other place than into your mouth. Go upstairs screaming, fly into a rage, and beat up your bed.

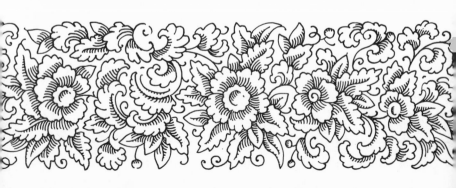

You're not hungry, you're anxious.

What is the thought that is making you anxious? Think it. Now stop thinking it.

Don't give it another thought.

Give your next thought to something that doesn't make you anxious.

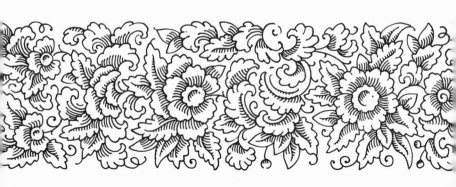

You want food.

Close your eyes.

Bring your awareness to your sphincter muscle.
Feel that you're contracting it. Now relax it. Feel
all your muscles begin to relax when you relax
your sphincter. With each exhalation of your
breath, keep relaxing .your sphincter.

Now you don't want food.

You have just solved the riddle of the Sphincter.

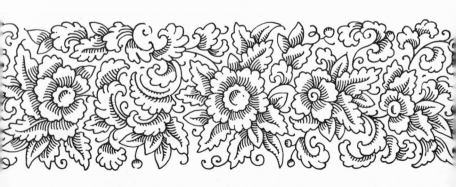

Food costs money. You are nibbling up your money. Stop nibbling and you will have more money.

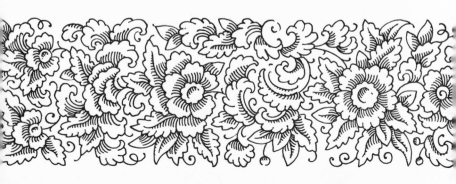

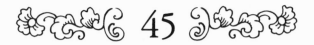

Put a chair next to the refrigerator. Re-route your habit of coming over to the refrigerator by sitting down in the chair. Relax. Take a break. Take a breather. Let your thoughts wander.

When you feel rested, get up and go away.

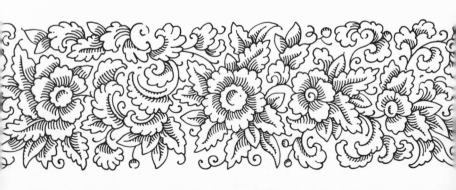

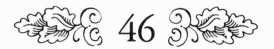

DON'T DO WHAT YOU'RE ABOUT TO DO!

CUT IT OUT!

DON'T BE STUPID!

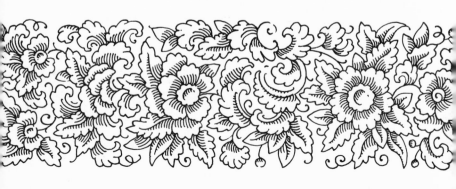

Identify the physical feeling that has led you to the refrigerator door. Name it. Did you call it hunger? Where is it? What does it feel like?

Is that hunger? Or is it heat and pressure?

Is it hunger or a small cramp?

That's not hunger. That's pain.

Go lie down and gently massage your stomach.

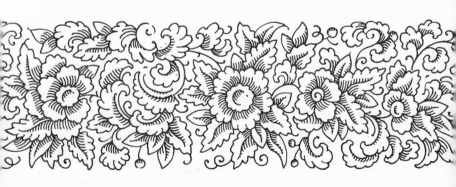

There *are* limits over you.

There are things you can do and things you can't do.

You can't nibble anymore. That's just true.

Welcome your limits. Limits don't constrain you, they protect you.

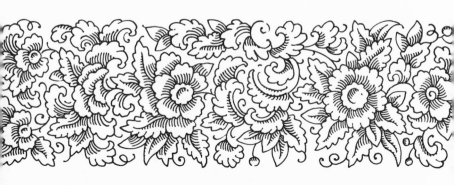

Remember that you have used your will in the past to undo other addictions. Remember that you have within you, *proven*, the power to control yourself. Just because your nibbling is a very difficult addiction, just because food and hunger are at the center of all addictions, still, nibbling is not an impossible addiction. There are no impossible addictions. The human will is stronger than any addiction.

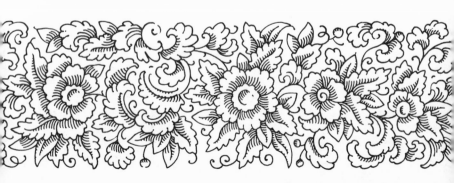

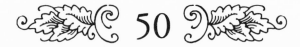

Sing the following Disco song. Make up your own tune and add verses using the names of your friends as you boogie-oogie-oogie yourself away from the refrigerator door.

Ask your bod', Todd.
It turns to gas, Cass.
What's a snack, Jack?
It's a nibble, Sybil.
Not the pita! Gita.
Just one serving, Irving.
You won't starve, Parv.
Use your willy, Billy.
It's just food-ith, Judith.
And it's insane, Jane.

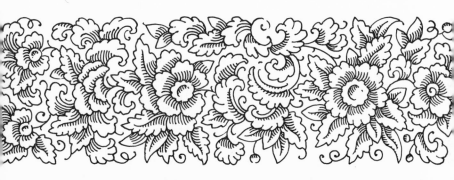

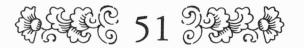

Move.

Take a walk. Ride a bike. Exercise. Dance.
Wrestle. Shake. Jog.

Run as fast as you can for as long as you can and
fall down exhausted.

Move!

Food doesn't want to come *into* you, energy wants
to come *out* of you.

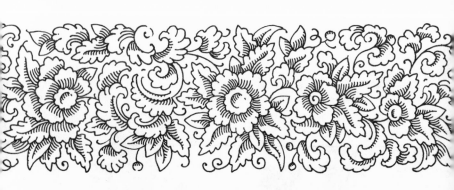

Stop saying, "It's hard."

"It's hard not to nibble."
"It's hard to get my food trip together."
"It's hard to lose weight."
"It's hard to walk away from this refrigerator."

If you say it's hard, it's hard.

Try saying, "It's easy."
Try saying, "It's a cinch."

In the beginning was the word.

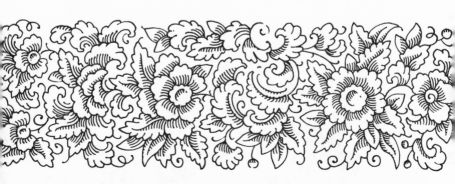

Close your eyes.

In your mind's eye, imagine that you are standing next to a person you hate. Now imagine that you suddenly assault and overpower this person, and you pry open the mouth of this person and begin to stuff food into it mercilessly. Really torture this person.

Keep cramming food down this person's mouth until this person blows up like a balloon and falls to the floor and dies at your feet.

Can you imagine that? Can you imagine hating someone that much?

Of course you can.

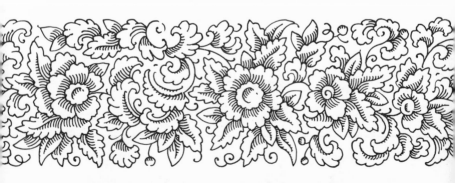

You hate yourself because all your life people called you bad. They called you naughty, selfish, whiny, lazy, loud, stubborn, stupid, mean, ugly, and fat. They thought you were bad. You believed them.

They were wrong.

You are good.

From the moment you were born until this moment as you stand at the refrigerator door, you have deserved unconditional love from everybody. Including yourself.

You can stop torturing this person now.

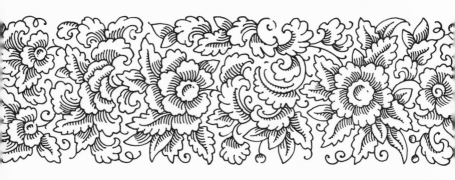

You are so obsessed with food that you are prone to interpret any bodily feeling as hunger. Check again. That's not your stomach, it's your bladder. It's full. Go pee.

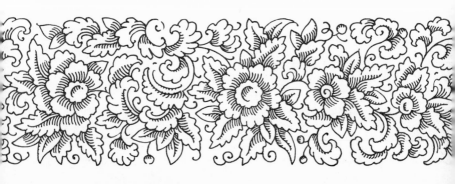

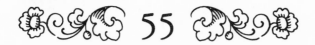

If you didn't nibble, your body would not have to work so hard digesting food. If your body didn't have to work so hard digesting food, you wouldn't be so tired. If you weren't so tired, you would need less sleep. If you needed less sleep, you would have more time. If you had more time, you wouldn't feel rushed and overburdened with things to do. If you didn't feel rushed and overburdened with things to do, you would feel peace.

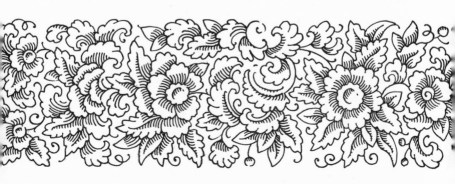

Your mouth wants food.

Now bring your awareness out of your mouth and into your stomach. Listen for the truth from your stomach. Don't trust your mouth. Think of the trouble your mouth has gotten you into in the past.

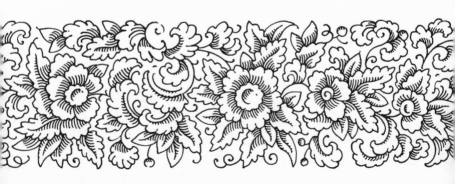

Wait. Just wait. Your hunger emerged. It will submerge. Something else will emerge. There's no emergency. Wait.

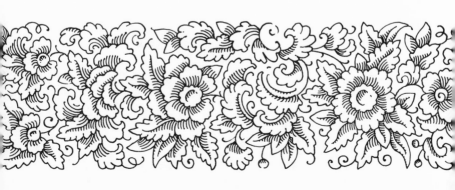

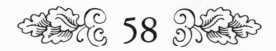

Go to a mirror and look in it. Say hello. Have a conversation with yourself. Let this conversation go where it will for as long as it wants. Enjoy your own company. You're not hungry, you're lonely.

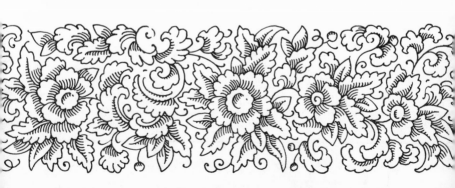

Before you go into the kitchen, plan your
passageway through.

"When I go into the kitchen, I will stop once,
at the sink, for water, and then leave."

Follow your plan.

Remember to make your plan before you enter the
kitchen, because once you're in the kitchen and
you see the food, all hell will break loose in your
eyeballs, and you will no longer be a reliable
planner.

Make plans for the next day as you lie in bed,
close to sleep, stuffed with food, slightly sick,
sincerely repentant, and clear as a bell.

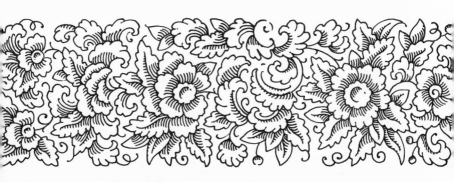

Sigh.

Keep sighing.

Stand right there at the refrigerator door sighing because you're sad that this time you can't open it. Cry if you need to.

It's a sad occasion. A loss. You're saying goodbye to something that was a comfort and a friend to you. Now life is calling you away. Goodbye, dear friend.

As you walk away from the refrigerator door, look back, like Ingrid Bergman at Humphrey Bogart in the fog in *Casablanca*, and sadly wave goodbye.

You came over to the refrigerator for a taste of something.

Now bring your awareness from your sense of taste to your sense of smell. Imagine the smell of the food you are about to taste. Close your eyes and imagine breathing it in through your nose. The food smells good. You feel pleasure.

Now open the refrigerator door and get the food you came over to taste, and put it in front of you. Bend down and inhale the aroma. Breathe it in. Imagine that you are being ethereally fed through your nose. There is no reason to experience your sense of taste because there is nourishment and deliciousness in your sense of smell.

Now put the food back and close the refrigerator.

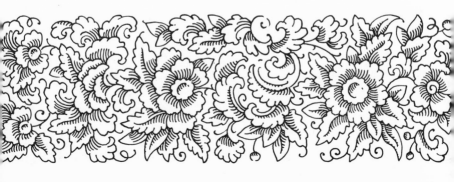

If you couldn't smell a thing, that's because you are stuffed with mucus from your constant nibbling. Some people call this condition a cold. Some people call it sinusitis or the flu. Some people call it nasal, and some people call it normal. Whatever you call it, you have no sense of smell.

Become aware that you have sacrificed one of your senses to your nibbling.

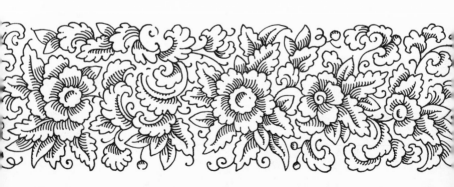

Ask yourself, "What is the thing I need to do right now in order not to have this nibble?"

When you hear it, do it.

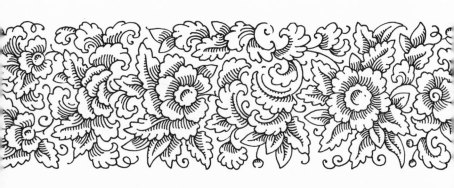

Close your eyes. Breathe.

In your mind's eye, begin to see all the foods you find delicious passing by you on an endless buffet table. Imagine the smell and taste of each dish as it passes before your eyes. Have a piece. Grab a bite. Go "Yum," and rub your tummy. Eat whatever you want for as long as you want and enjoy yourself.

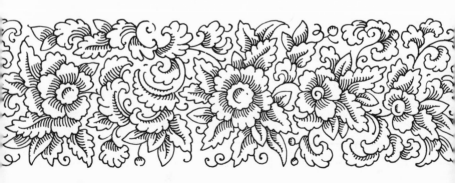

You're not hungry, you're afraid.

An instant ago, a thought came into your head that made you afraid. Like everybody else, you're afraid of being afraid, so you're over here at the refrigerator about to throw food on top of your fear.

Go back one instant. What was the thought that came into your head that made you afraid? Look straight at it. It's a scary thought.

It's okay to be afraid.

You're *still* not breathing.

Take a deep breath.

Breathe.

The feeling that brought you to the refrigerator
door is a feeling. Big deal. What's a feeling?

Feelings come and feelings go.

Close your eyes.

Imagine that you are standing on the bank of a
river. See the river. This river is the river of your
feelings. Watch your feelings as they float by you
on the river. Watch the river. Don't jump in.

When the feeling that brought you to the
refrigerator door floats by, watch it pass.

It takes energy to nibble, and it takes energy to digest what you nibble. All the energy that you give to your nibbling could be going elsewhere. It could be going to the world. There's unspeakable suffering out there, and your energy is needed immediately.

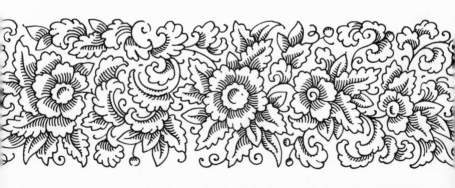

If you must nibble, if you absolutely *must*, think about nibbling something heavy, cooked, starchy, soft, fatty, greasy, sweet, salted, and dead, with artificial preservatives and lots of chemicals.

Now get nauseous.

Now think about nibbling something raw, fresh, juicy, and alive.

Now get an apple.

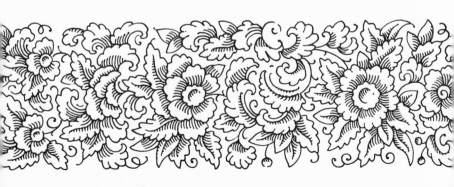

Go to the telephone. Call a friend. Tell your
friend of your struggles at the refrigerator door.
Ask your friend for help; support; encouragement;
appreciation; inspiration; love; the truth; some
humor; compassionate understanding.

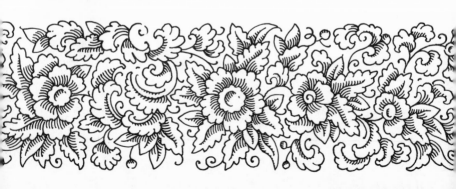

Pause for a moment. Then, throwing your hands up in the air, exclaim, "Oh *no*! Stuffing your face *AGAIN*?!"

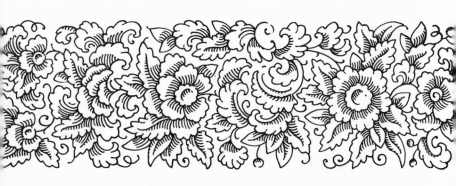

Become aware that you are tense. You are either tensely nibbling, or tensely about to nibble, or tensely standing in front of the refrigerator deciding whether to nibble. Feel your tension.

Feel it once and for all. Become completely tense and tight.

Now relax.

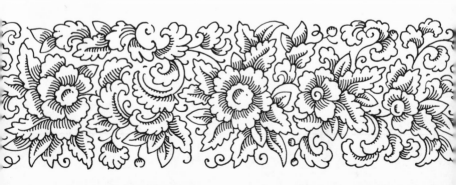

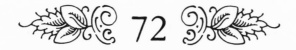

From meal to meal, fast. Call it a fast. It is easier to fast than not to nibble.

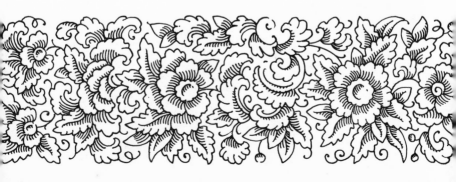

The absolute worst thing that could happen to you from your nibbling is that you would put such an outrageous burden on your body with food that your body would become exhausted, give up, decide to die, and develop a horrible degenerative disease from which you would die in agony.

That's the absolute worst.

If that happens, you would no longer be struggling with your attachment to food, you would be struggling with your attachment to life, so choose your struggle.

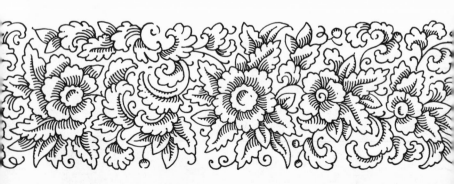

If you need to walk through the kitchen, walk through the kitchen with your eyes down. If you're standing at the refrigerator door, keep your eyes down. If you open the door, keep your eyes down. There's nothing there. Close the door. Don't look. Your eyes get you in trouble all the time.

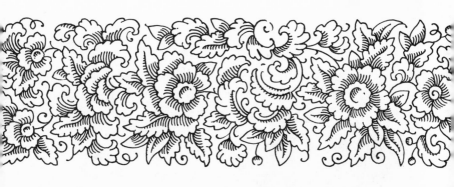

You're hungry. Hunger is a feeling. Bring your awareness to the feeling. Feel it. Is it *so* bad? It's just another feeling that comes and goes and means you no harm.

Do you think that if you have this nibble, your hunger will not come back?

Hang out with your hunger. Make it your friend. Enjoy the afternoon together.

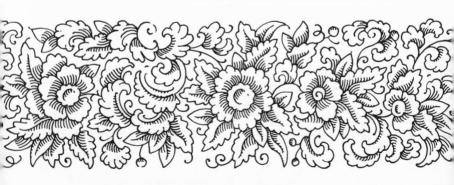

Grind yourself to a screeching halt with the emergency brake of absolute moral courage.

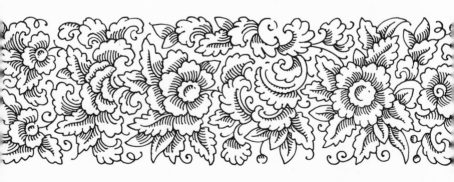

You are standing at the refrigerator door and there are other people in the kitchen. There are other eyes besides your own in the room and everybody is watching. Even if they don't look like they're watching, they're watching. Everybody is watching everything all the time.

You don't want to be seen doing in public what you do in private. It's slightly shameful.

Accept their eyes as a gift to help you control yourself this time. *Use* your shame Don't be so proud that you won't use even your shame as a tool.

Remember to drop the tool when you're done with it. Leave your shame at the refrigerator door, and replace it with triumph as you walk back into everybody's eyes.

Drop the image of yourself as a nibbler. The image creates the reality. You permit yourself to be what you imagine yourself to be.

Imagine yourself to be a non-nibbler.

What would a non-nibbler do at the refrigerator door?

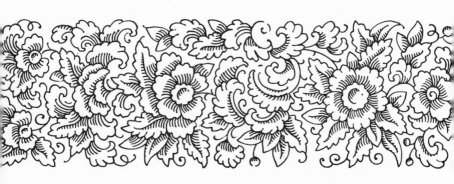

Feel the juices moving around in your stomach.
You think they mean hunger, so you came over to
the refrigerator to nibble.

But they don't mean hunger.

They mean that the last time you ate, you overate,
and you paralyzed your digestive juices for hours.

That's not hunger, that's your stomach coming out
of a coma.

Put one of the following signs on the refrigerator door.

STOP

BEAR LEFT

NO ENTRANCE

NO EXIT

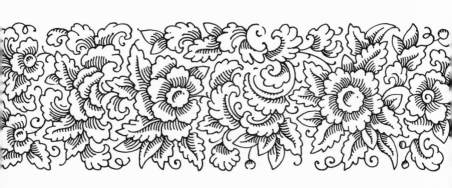

When an addiction is broken, agony is released into your system, and you have to feel it for a time. Be prepared for some agony when you stop your nibbling. Say yes to the agony. It is not so awful an agony as you think, and it has an end. Nibbling is agony without end.

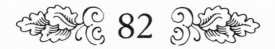

Remember that you not only *have* a body, you *are* a body. When you nibble, you are that which is doing, and that which is done to. You are the victimizer, and you are the victim.

Plead with yourself.

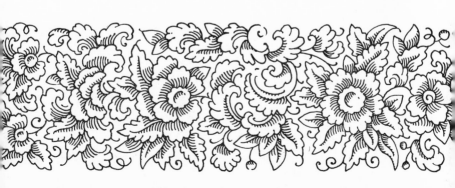

Do you remember the starving people your mother used to tell you about to get you to eat more?

They're still starving.

Millions of people are starving on this earth.

So eat less.

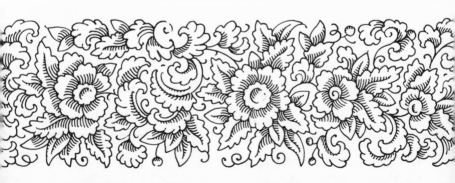

Stop. Close your eyes.

From your heart call for your guardian angel to come down and take you gently by the shoulder and bring you back to safety.

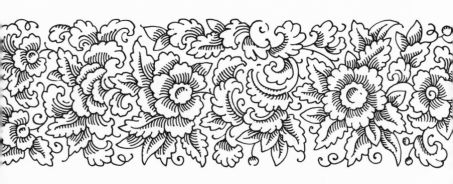

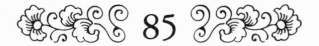

Chant the following out loud:

> I *am digging my grave with my teeth.*
> I *am digging my grave with my teeth.*
> I *am digging my grave with my teeth.*
> I *am digging my grave with my teeth.*

This is a very effective chant, especially if visualized.

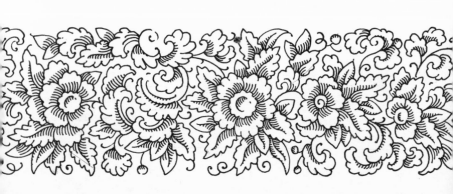

As you stand at the refrigerator door, ask yourself, "What lie am I going to tell myself *this* time to justify my nibbling?"

When you hear it, congratulate yourself for your creative thinking, and laugh.

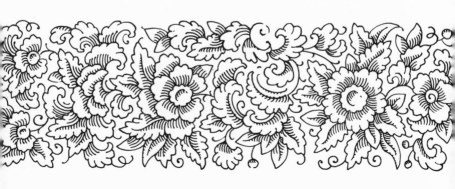

If you open the refrigerator door and you choose to nibble this time, all is not lost.

Practice Right Nibbling.

Take a breath. Become quiet inside. Reach for your food calmly and prepare it with care. Go slow. Sit down. Give thanks. Chew well. Put your utensil down between each bite. Breathe. Enjoy. Be aware of what you are doing.

What you are doing is eating.

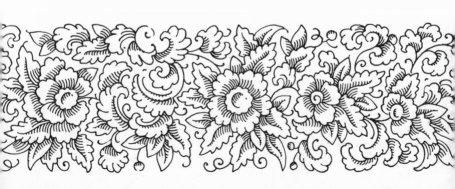

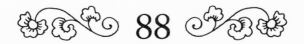

When you were an infant, you were powerless to bring food to yourself when hungry, so when you got hungry, you got scared. You didn't know if food was coming. You were scared you would starve to death.

And now you're here at the refrigerator, still scared you'll starve to death, and about to cram food into your mouth as fast as you can.

Stop. Remember that you're not powerless anymore. You're a grown-up now. You're in charge, and you can bring food to yourself whenever you want. Remind yourself that there is definitely food in your immediate future.

And wait for it. Wait for a meal. Make it a scrumptious meal. Make it a meal worth waiting for.

The meal is the reward.

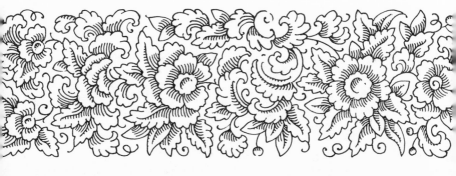

You were at ease. Then you felt dis-ease. Then you came over to the refrigerator.

Now you are standing at the refrigerator transforming your dis-ease into disease through the medium of food.

Remember that you can transform your dis-ease back into ease through the medium of breath.

Breathe.

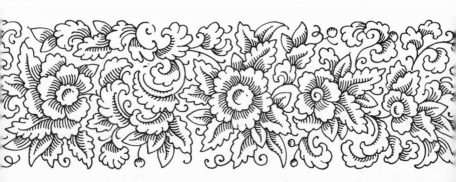

Give yourself orders.

If you don't like giving yourself orders, or if you never take your own orders, ask a friend to do it for you.

> "Jane, before you go, tell me what to do this morning."
> "Robert, don't nibble. I'll see you at lunch."
> "Thank you, Jane."

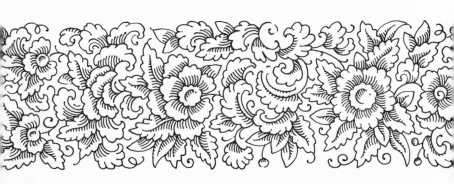

Stop living in the past. Your idea that you can still maintain this habit and get away with it is foolishness. It's over. You don't want it to be over, but it is.

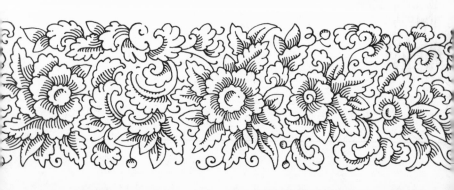

Put a mirror near your refrigerator. As you are about to nibble, look at the mirror. See the face you wear when you nibble.

If you become ashamed of this face, feel the shame strongly and let it pull you away from the refrigerator.

Or try loving the face you see in the mirror. Forgive that face. You are doing your absolute best, every moment. Considering everything that has happened to you in your life, and the food hysteria you inherited from the culture you grew up in, it's a miracle you haven't eaten yourself to death long ago.

So love yourself. Love yourself for your strength, your courage, your patience, and your persistence.

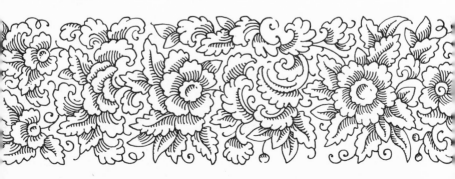

Love yourself for putting a mirror near the refrigerator.

After you have loved yourself for all your wonderful qualities, love yourself for all your terrible qualities. Love yourself for the weakness that brought you to the refrigerator.

Now, love yourself neither for your strength nor for your weakness, but just for yourself. You are. You deserve love.

If you are still looking in the mirror, you will notice that your face has changed.

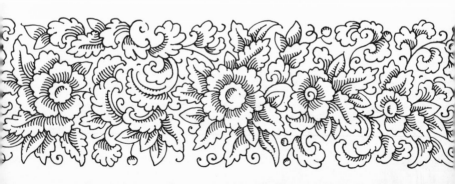

Fold your arms across your chest and say out loud, "No, I absolutely forbid it." Be very stern.

Now get angry and jump up and down screaming, "Yes! I want to! I want to!"

Who is saying "No"? And who is screaming "Yes!"? And who is that sneaking a nibble in between?

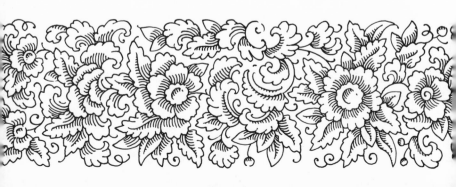

There's nowhere to go.

Nibble as much as you want, little mousekin, go
to every movie in town, have a drink, have a
smoke, get high, go up, go down, go shopping,
go around the world, have sex with everybody in
sight, search out every imaginable kind of
stimulation and sensation, and still, when it's
over, you'll come right back to yourself.

Just forget it. It's hopeless. Stay where you are and
be free.

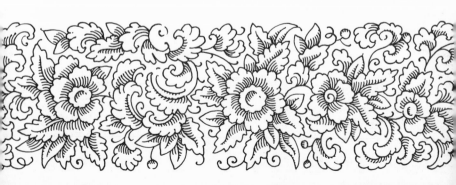

You'll feel better after you have this nibble.

No you won't.

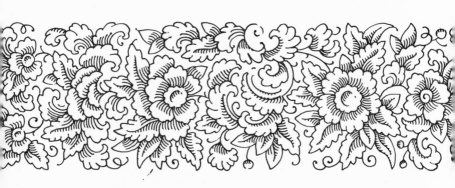

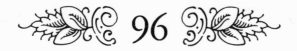

Coke is *not* the real thing. They're trying to confuse you. They're all trying to confuse you. Don't let them confuse you anymore. Find out what the real thing is.

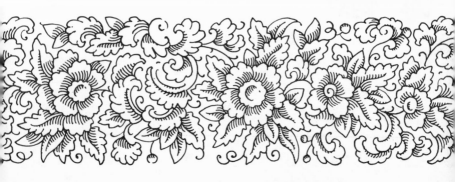

You are about to nibble. You reach for the refrigerator door. You reach for the food. You are reaching. You are reaching outward.

Now close your eyes and reach inward.

It's in *there*, silly.

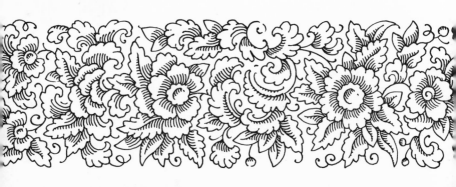

Standing at the refrigerator door, your hand on the handle, ask your inner self out loud, "Do you want to have this nibble?"

Then, in a different voice, ask, "Who do you want to talk to in here?"

Then ask, "Who are *you?*"

Then ask, "Who is asking?"

Then walk away from the refrigerator scratching your head.

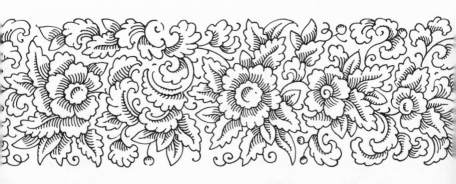

Imagine that when you open the refrigerator door
what you will see will be the horribly grotesque
face of a hideous monster staring straight back at
you. You will die from sheer fright when you see
this face. That's who's behind the refrigerator
door.

Really.

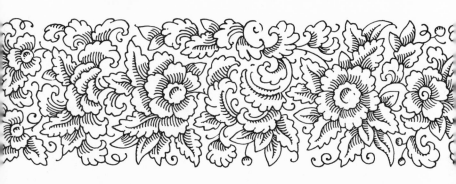

The table of the Lord is an altar, and who eats at the table of the Lord is in a temple. Enter only into the Lord's temple when you feel in yourselves the call of the Lord's angels, for all that you eat in sorrow, or in anger, or without desire, becomes a poison in your body.

Jesus of Nazareth, *The Essene Gospel of Peace*

Become aware that every living thing in the whole wide world is watching you right now and time has stopped.

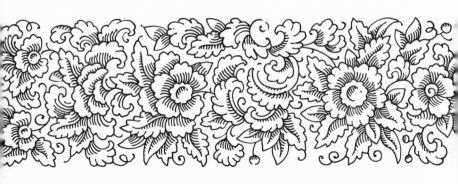

You experience your hunger as pain. You experience your nibbling as pleasure. Pain and pleasure, pain and pleasure. It is an endlessly turning wheel, and you are tied to it.

But at the center of the wheel, not turning, completely still, is a place where you understand the illusion of pain and pleasure, you understand that they are one.

The ride up is the ride down.

So why take the ride?

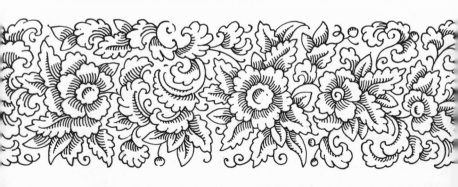

Sit down. Think it over.

Change your mind.

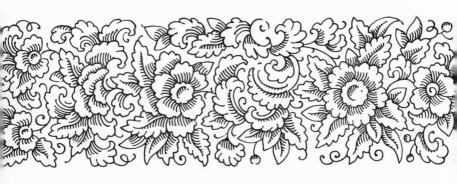

Become aware that you have a craving for food right now.

Now see this craving as something you *have*, not as something you are. Imagine that you are actually holding this craving in your hand.

Now put this craving for food in a specially marked jar labeled "Cravings for Food," which you keep in the kitchen near the refrigerator.

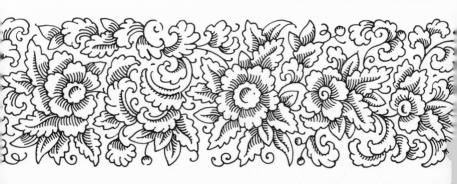

Feel the uselessness of all action. It's really hopeless. There's no reason to nibble. There's no reason not to nibble. There's no reason to do anything. Everything changes and nothing changes. It doesn't matter *what* you do. You might as well die.

Feel that despair. Stand on that precipice.

Now jump from that precipice to perfect serenity—because there's nowhere else to go.

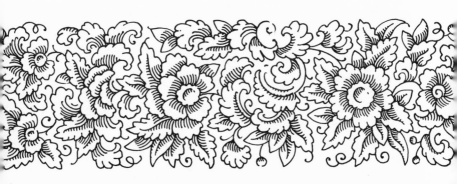

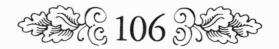

You're free. No one's over you now. The battle is won. You can do what you want. What do you want?

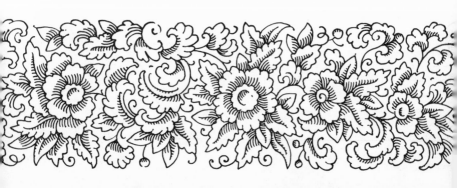

Stop. Look around you.

As you look around, become aware that there is a
world of sense objects out there coming to you
through your eyes. Your eyes are attached to these
sense objects. And you are attached to your eyes.

Now break the attachment. You are not your eyes.
You are watching from within. Your eyes are
looking around you, but you are watching from
within.

Now open the refrigerator door and behold the
food. Stay within. Be undisturbed. Just look.
Close the door.

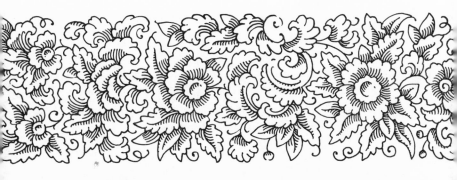

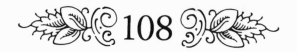

You're not running things. You're not making a single decision in your life. You are engaged in activity, but you're not acting. Everything is just happening and you're along for the ride. The ride took you here to the refrigerator, and now it's taking you back again, and you can't do a damn thing about it.

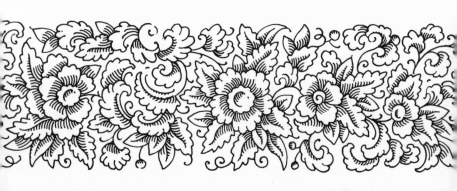

Close your eyes, go inside, and bring your
attention to your heart.

Now open your heart to the love inside you, and
breathe the love in and out of your heart. With
each breath let love pour through you. You love
the food. You love yourself. You love everything.

The thing that you were about to do, to the food
and to yourself, is filled with hate.

But you are now filled with love. You *are* love.
You can do no harm, and nibbling is harm.

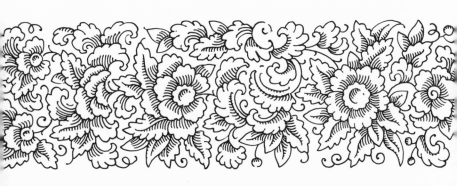

Your children are watching.

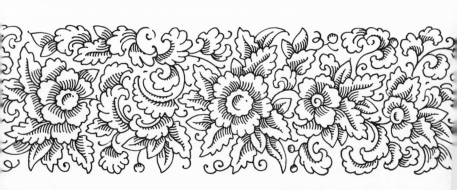

Decide.
The debate stops when you decide.
The debate is the suffering.
Stop the debate.

Set a goal.

"I will treat my body with respect and care."
"I will use my energy to become great at my
    vocation."
"I will become a model of health and happiness
    to all around me."
"I will help heal the earth by healing myself."

Listen to the voice of your goal above the clamor
of your other voices calling for a nibble. Derive
the discipline you need to not nibble by becoming
a disciple of your goal.

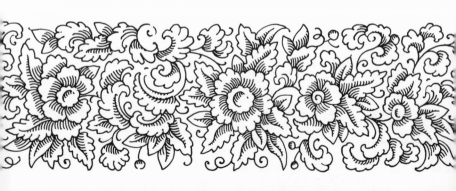

Read these words by Mahatma Gandhi.

The Gita* *enjoins not temperance in food but "meagerness." Meagerness is a perpetual fast. Meagerness means just enough to sustain the body for the service for which it is made.*

Voluntary meager eating is one of the most difficult things in the world. Meager food voluntarily taken must *lead to perfect poise, i.e., perfect health of body and mind. We can but make the attempt.*

Now try to think of a reason why Mahatma Gandhi would lie to you.

* *The Bhagavad-gītā* (*The Song of God*), the sacred gospel of Hinduism.

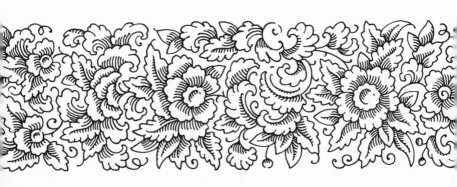

Imagine that someone is dreaming this whole scene. Everything—the refrigerator, the food inside it, your desire for the food, you, these words, this moment—it's all a dream.

And you're the dreamer.

Dream that you walk away from the refrigerator.

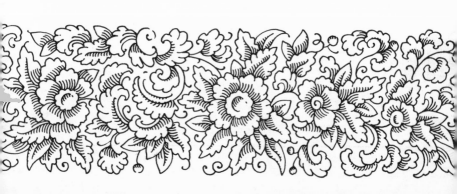

Stop. Close your eyes.

Become aware that you have a body. Feel the
sensation of being inside this body. Feel the air as
it gently presses against your skin. Feel your feet
where they touch the floor. Now breathe, and
experience your breath coming in and going out of
you.

There is an inside, there is an outside. There is
you, there is not you.

Now let the boundaries of your body begin to
dissolve, and you begin to merge with everything
around you. Expand. Melt. Expand. Expand.

Now there is no outside. Everything is inside.
You are everything.

Nibble?

But everything is inside.

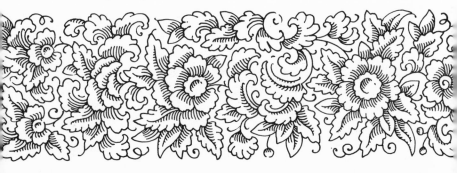

Grace is trying to pull you up. Gravity is trying to pull you down. Which way is the refrigerator?

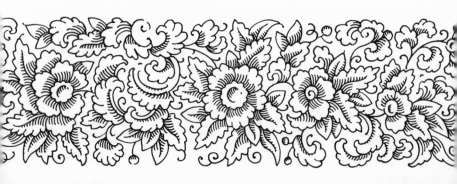

It will feel good to have this nibble. It really will. It will feel like a rush, an ecstasy, a delightful little trip outside yourself.

And then the little trip will be over.

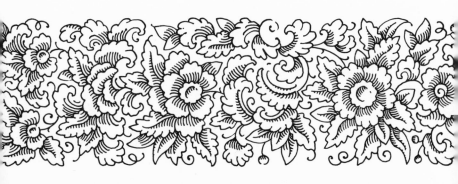

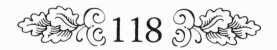

With all the force of your will, no matter what you're feeling or how bad the agony, break the addiction right now and say "No."

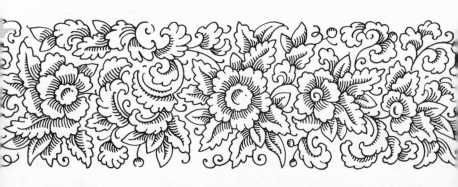

And if not now, when?

Hillel, *Pirke Aboth (Ethics of the Fathers)*

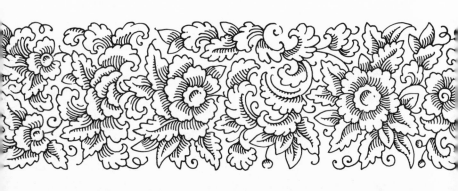

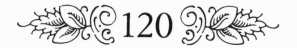

Spit it out.

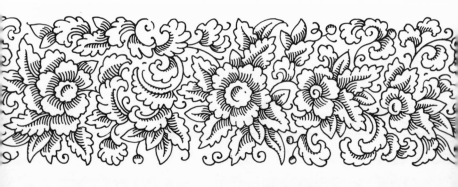

You love your family. You love your friends. You love all people.

They are hurting themselves with their nibbling. They are killing themselves. They need your help.

They need your example.

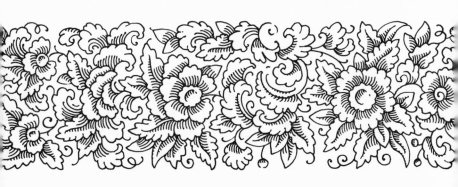

Imagine that the act of eating is a holy ritual.
Imagine that your refrigerator is a temple.
Imagine that you are a worshiper who has come to
this temple.

Imagine that everything is holy.

What are you doing?

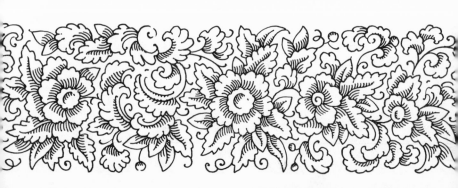

Pray fervently.

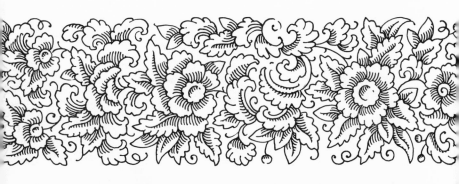

Believe that you can stop nibbling. Believe that
The No-Nibbling Book can help you, and use it.

"I'll believe it when I see it."

Nope.

You'll see it when you believe it.

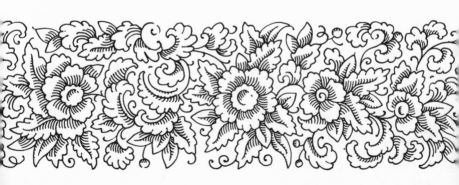

"I'm a bad person and bad things are going to happen to me and everything is going to get worse and the world is coming to an end."

That's fear.

"I'm a good person and good things are going to happen to me and everything is going to get better and Heaven is coming to Earth."

That's excitement.

Nibbling is the lid you put on the fear, and fear is the lid you put on the excitement.

Now take off the lids and uncover the excitement. The excitement is uncontainable. The excitement is the truth.

Standing at the refrigerator door, begin jumping up and down clapping your hands together and singing, "I'm so excited! I'm so excited!"

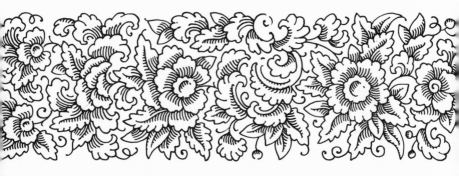

Breathe.

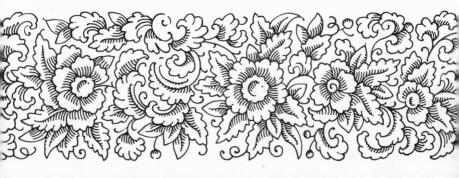

Meditate.

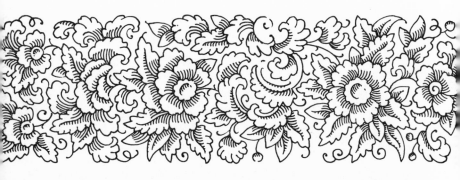

Use any one of these techniques.

Use a combination of these techniques.

Use all of these techniques simultaneously.

Afterword

The Earth is being healed. Despite appearances, the process that is happening to the Earth is a healing process.

You are part of the Earth. You are being healed. The process that is happening to you is a healing process.

It is happening. Light and love and joy and health are coming. They are coming within you and without you, at the right speed, in their own time.

So have no fear.

To everything there is a season, and a time for every purpose under the heaven.

When the time comes for your nibbling to stop, your nibbling will stop. At the right time, it will just drop away.

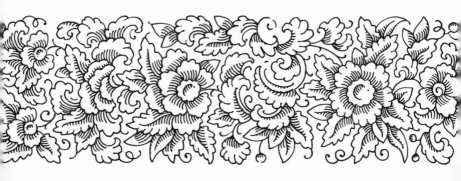

Is this the right time?

Yes, but don't worry about it.

It's a process. You will do your best. Be proud of yourself. Be patient with yourself. Forgive yourself, and begin again.

Trust the process.

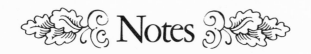# Notes

Number 13: *Voices of Wisdom: Jewish Ideals and Ethics for Everyday Living* by Francis Klagsbrun, New York: Pantheon Books, 1980, pp. 213, 214.

Number 100: *The Essene Gospel of Peace*, Szekely, Edmond Bordeaux, trans., Academy Books, 3085 Reynard Way, San Diego, California 92103, pp. 55–56.

Number 113: *Less Is More: The Art of Voluntary Poverty*, VandenBroeck, Goldian, ed., Harper & Row, 1978, pp. 259, 262.

Number 119: *Pirke Aboth*, Chapter I, Mishnah 14, translated and annotated by Hyman E. Goldin, New York: Hebrew Publishing Company, 1962, p. 12.